Joey Discovers:
He Has Worm Poop On His Teeth!

By Dr. R. Anthony Matheny

A Story to Motivate Kids about the Importance of Brushing and Flossing

Copyright © 2013 Dr. R. Anthony Matheny
All rights reserved.

ISBN: 149366185X
ISBN-13: 9781493661855

Joey Discovers:

HE HAS WORM POOP ON HIS TEETH!

A story to motivate kids about the importance of brushing and flossing

By
Dr. R. Anthony Matheny

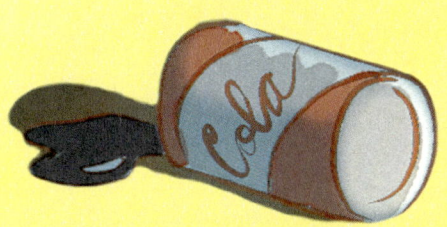

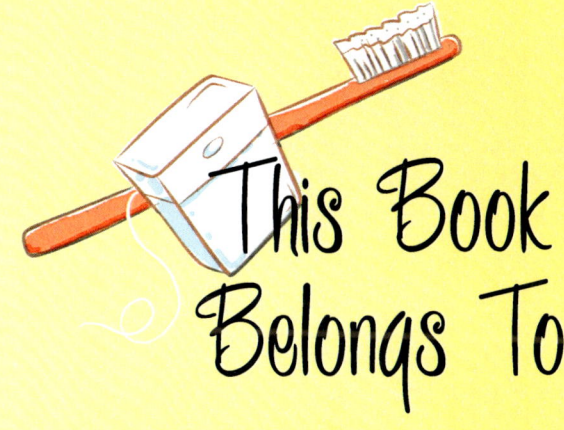

_____

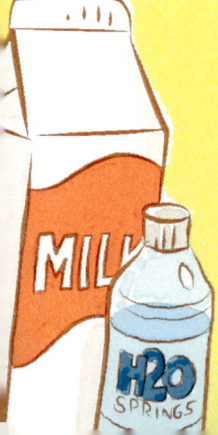

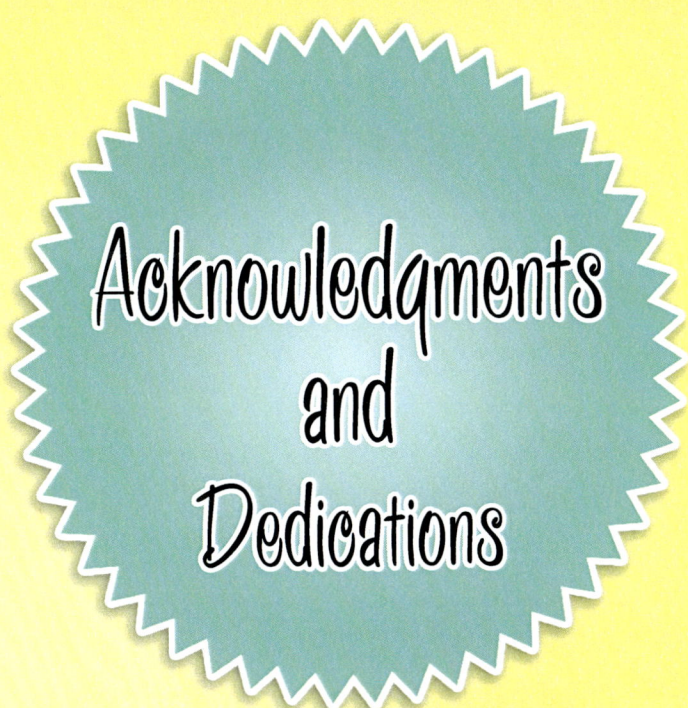

Acknowledgments and Dedications

This book is dedicated to my wife, Kathy, and son, Collin, who encouraged me to put this motivating story to print to help kids everywhere realize the importance of brushing and flossing.

I would like to acknowledge Dr. James Strawn, a great friend and dentist whom I heard tell an abbreviated version of this story to children he treated. It helped to motivate kids in his office to brush better and now it's helping children worldwide.

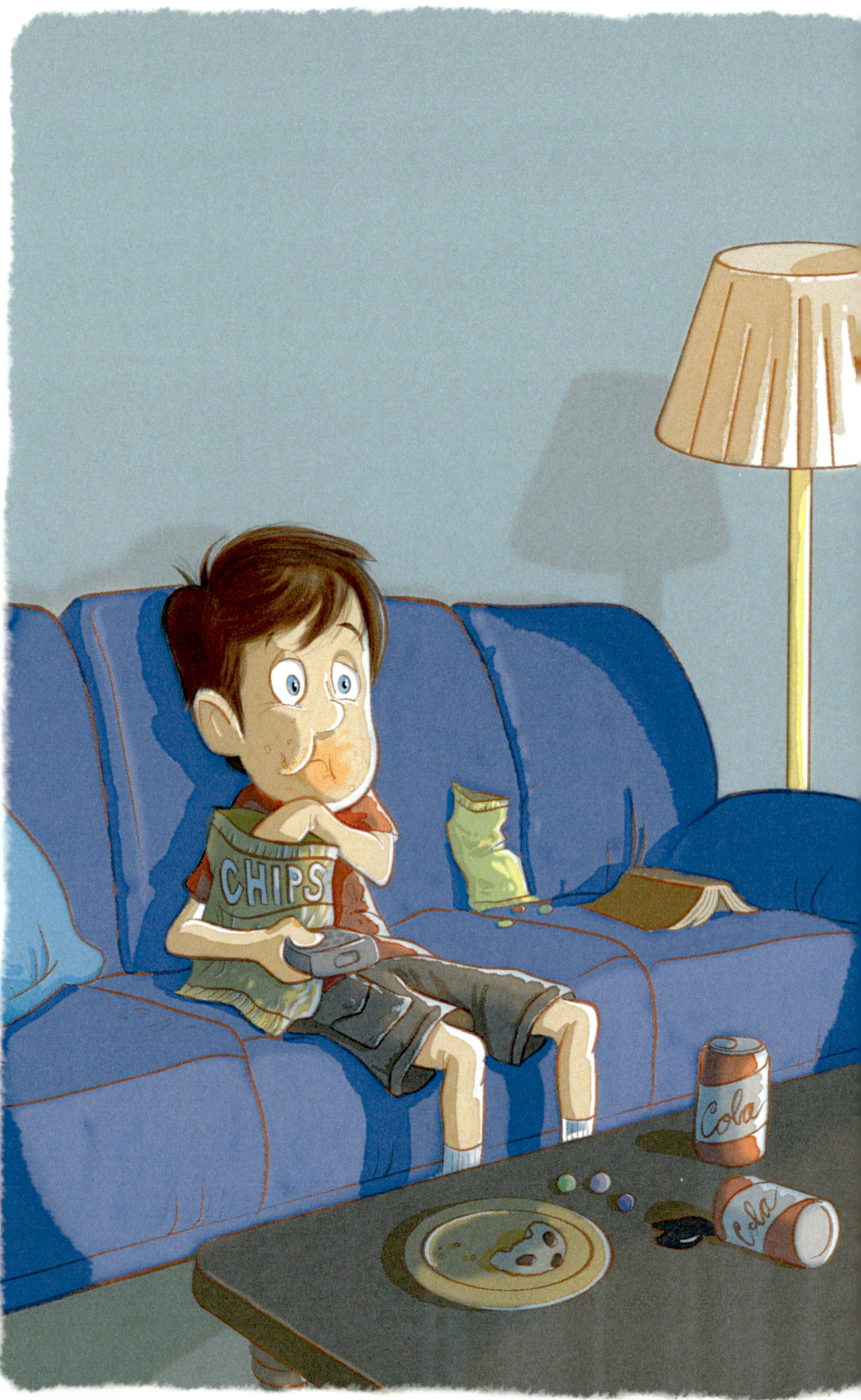

Joey was a third grade student at Jensen Beach Elementary in Florida. He was like most nine-year-old kids. He enjoyed hanging out with his friends, watching television, and playing video games.

He also enjoyed his snacks and drinks, like candy and candy bars, soda pop, milk, and juice. These all have a lot of sugar in them, but all Joey knew was that they tasted great.

Joey's mom, Kathy, always told him, "Joey, go brush your teeth!"

Joey whined back, "Awww, Mom, do I really have to? I brushed yesterday."

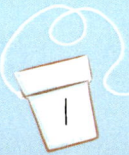

"Yes, Joey, you have to brush at least twice a day, especially after having sugary snacks," Kathy reminded him.

This went on for weeks. Kathy kept asking, "Joey, did you brush your teeth before bed? Joey, did you brush before going to school? Joey, did you brush after eating that candy?"

And Joey would answer, "What's the big deal, anyway?"

"Well, Joey, you don't want to get cavities, do you?" His mom would say.

Joey wanted to know what a cavity was. His mom tried to explain that it was a hole in your tooth and if you got a cavity, you had to go to the dentist to get it fixed. This answered Joey's question, but it still did not make Joey want to brush his teeth. He thought of it as a chore that he had to do, but didn't want to.

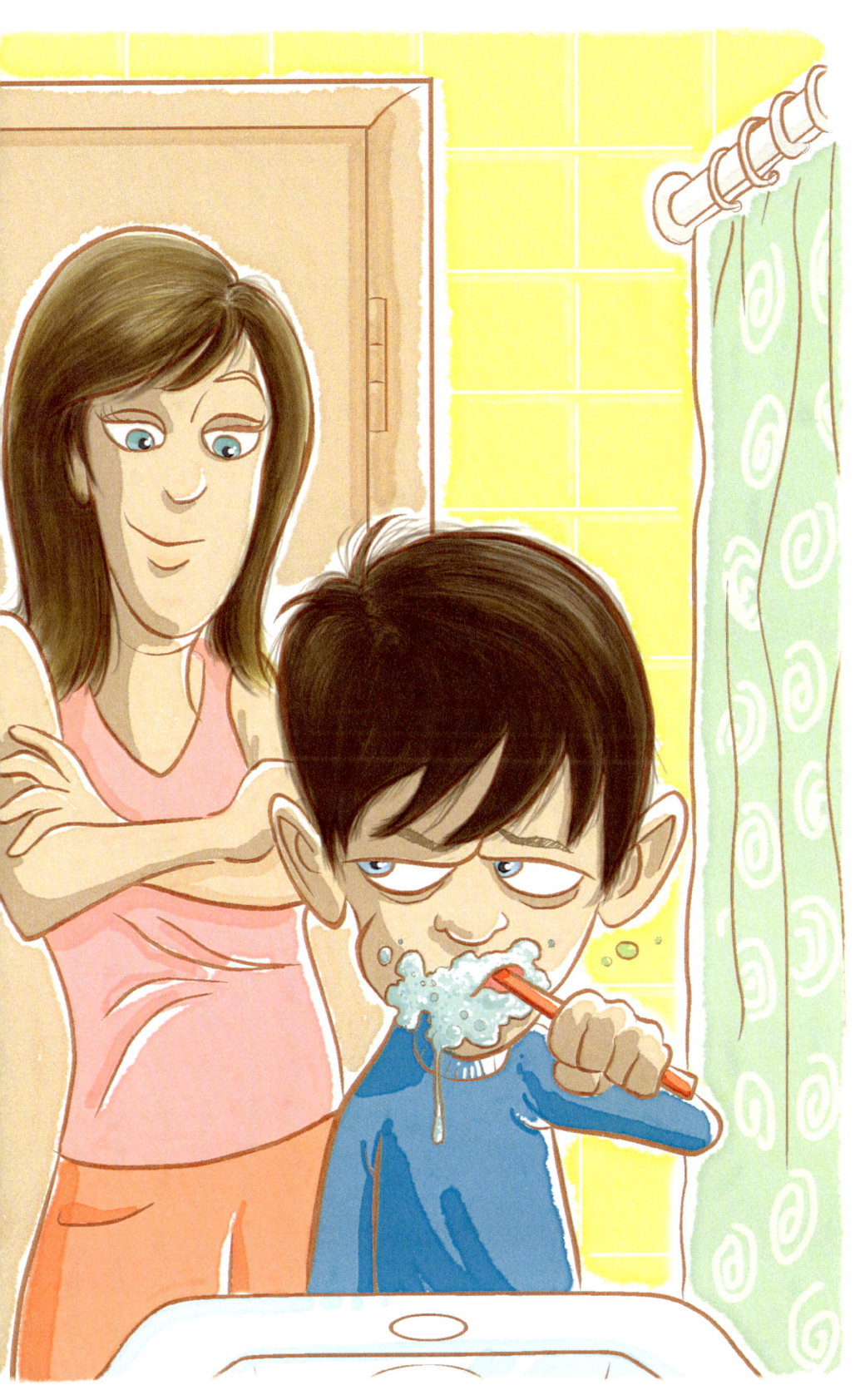

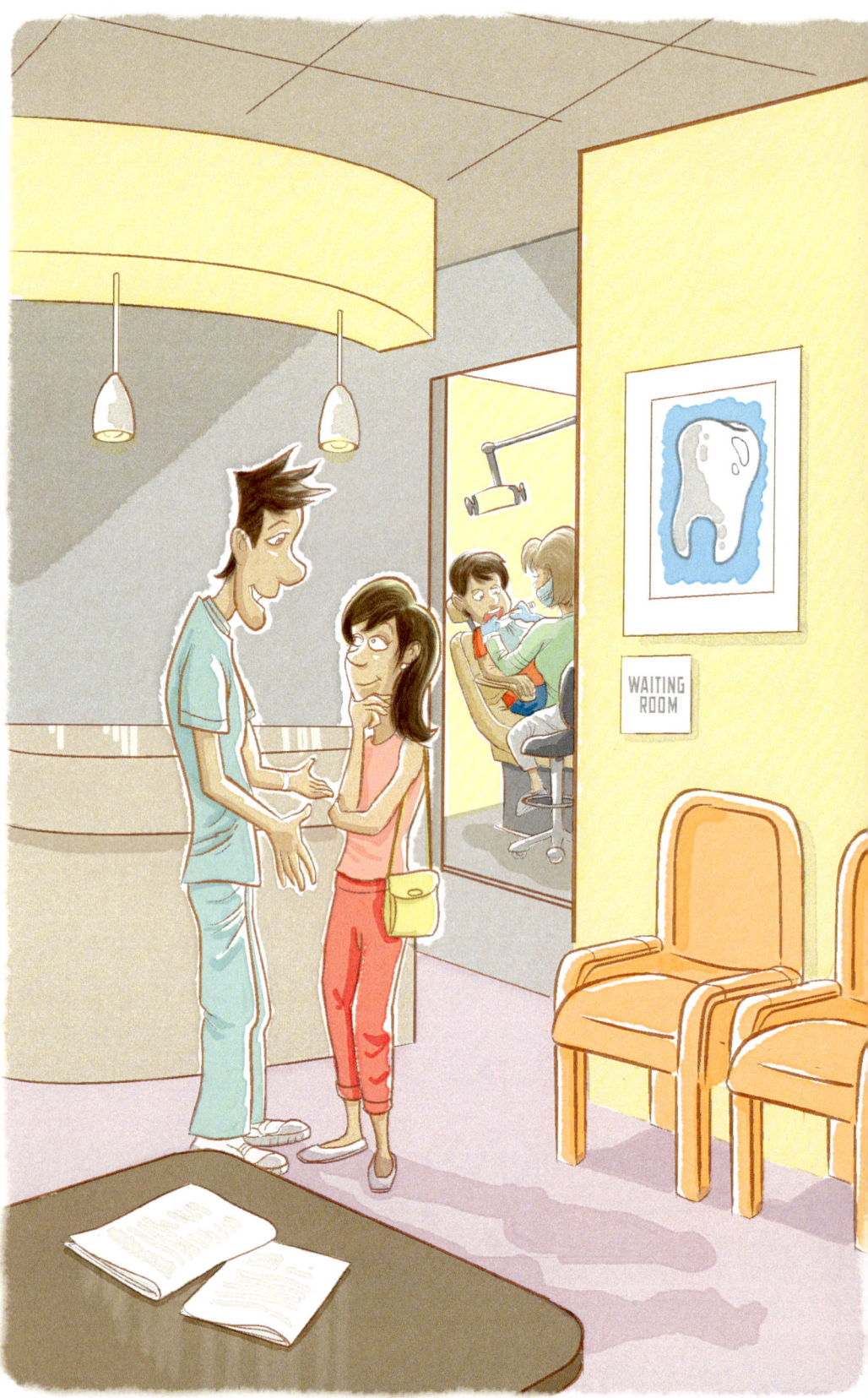

The next week, Joey had an appointment with his dentist, Dr. Tony, to have his teeth cleaned and checked. Kathy took Joey to Dr. Tony's office. While a nice dental hygienist cleaned his teeth, Dr. Tony came out to the waiting room to say hello to Kathy.

Kathy explained to Dr. Tony that she was having a really hard time getting Joey to brush and floss. She told him how she was always nagging him to do it.

"I have some free time after Joey's teeth are cleaned," said Dr. Tony. "Why don't I tell him a story that has really helped other kids realize the importance of brushing and flossing?"

"That would be great!" exclaimed Kathy.

Once the dental hygienist was done, Dr. Tony went into the room to check Joey's teeth. He noticed that Joey's gums were more red than usual and that he had a couple of cavities that needed to be fixed. Dr. Tony could tell that Joey was not brushing as well or as often as he should.

"Joey, let me tell you a story that may help you keep your teeth clean," said Dr. Tony.

"Okay," said Joey, wondering what Dr. Tony could tell him that would ever make him want to brush his teeth.

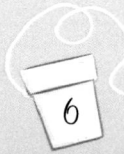

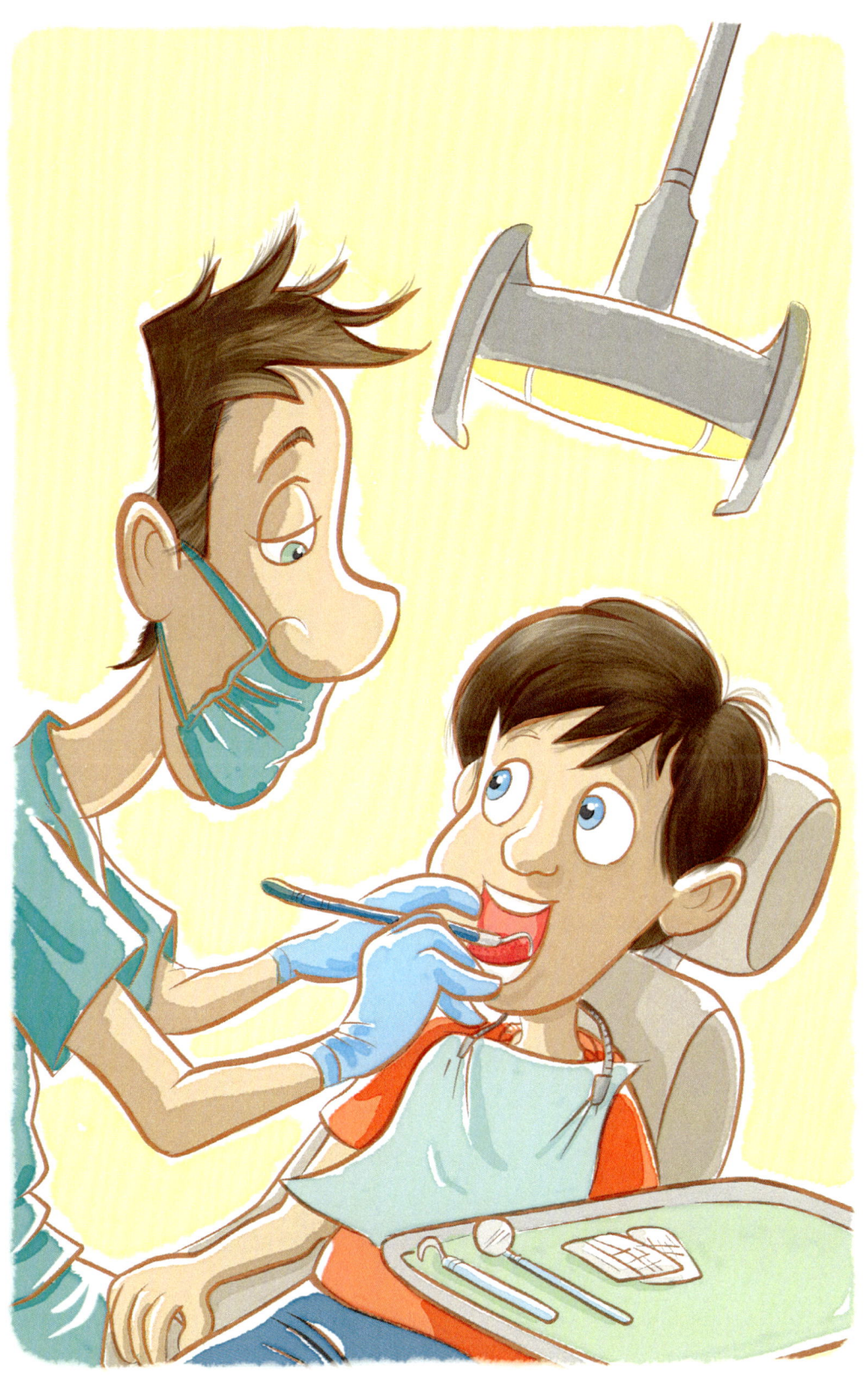

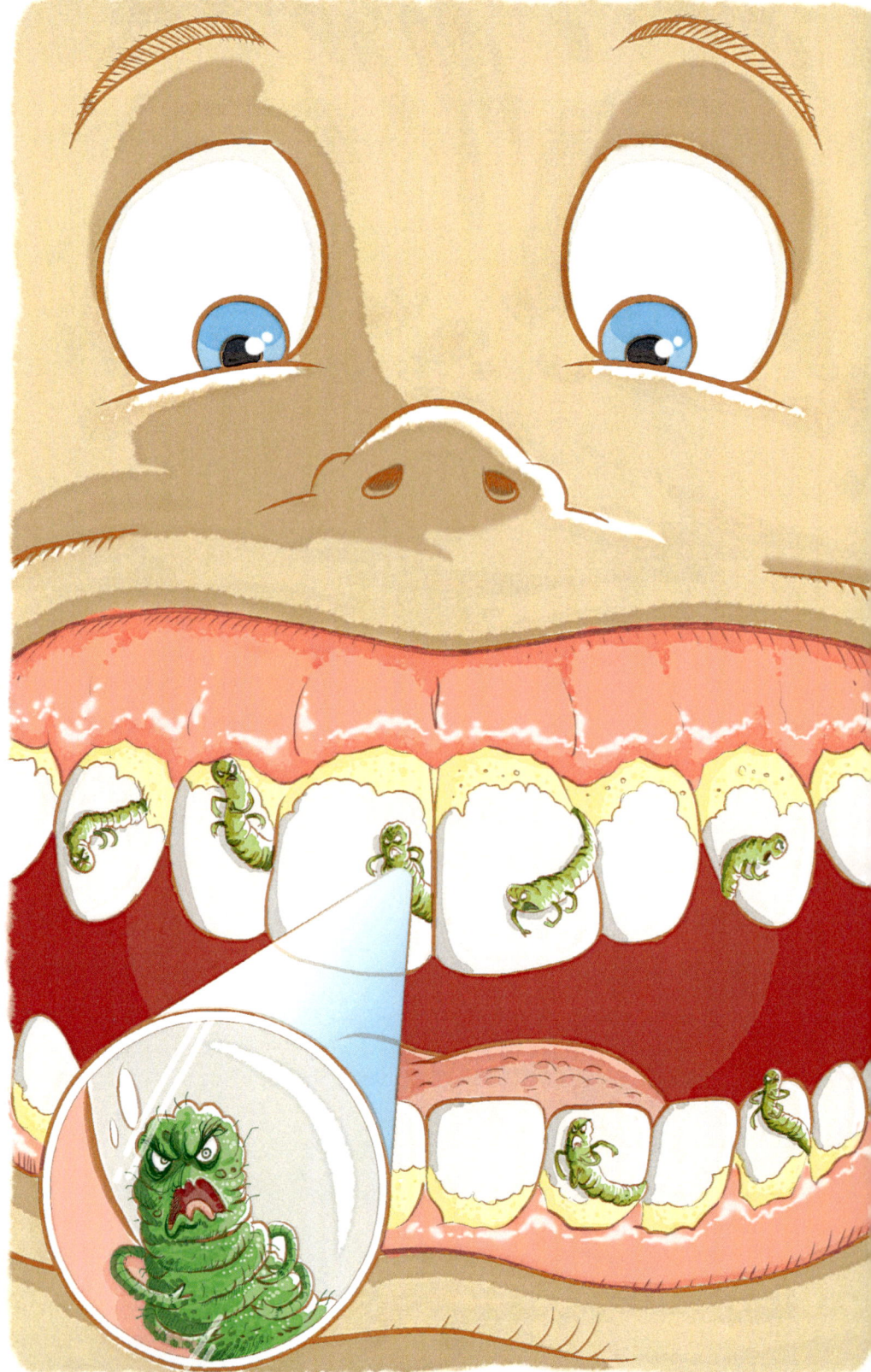

"You see, Joey," said Dr. Tony, "everybody's mouth has teeth, gums, lips, and a tongue. But there's something else in your mouth that you cannot see with your eyes. They are called bacteria, and they are germs that live in everyone's mouths. If you look at the germs under a microscope, they look like little worms."

Joey was shocked. "You mean I have worms in my mouth?" he asked.

"Very small ones, but yes, you do," Dr. Tony replied.

"Gross!" Joey yelled.

"Well, Joey, it actually gets worse. Along with those worms, you also have worm poop on your teeth!" Dr. Tony said.

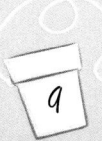

Joey couldn't believe what he just heard. "No way, that's disgusting!" Joey said loudly.

"Tell me, Joey," Dr. Tony said, "where do you go after you eat or drink a lot?"

"To the bathroom," Joey said.

"That's right," said Dr. Tony. "The worms live in our mouths, so where do you think they go to the bathroom after they eat?"

Joey thought for a second and then answered, "In our mouths?"

"That's right," said Dr. Tony. "In our mouths and on our teeth, gums, and tongue!"

"That's sick!" Joey said with an awful look on his face.

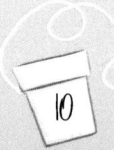

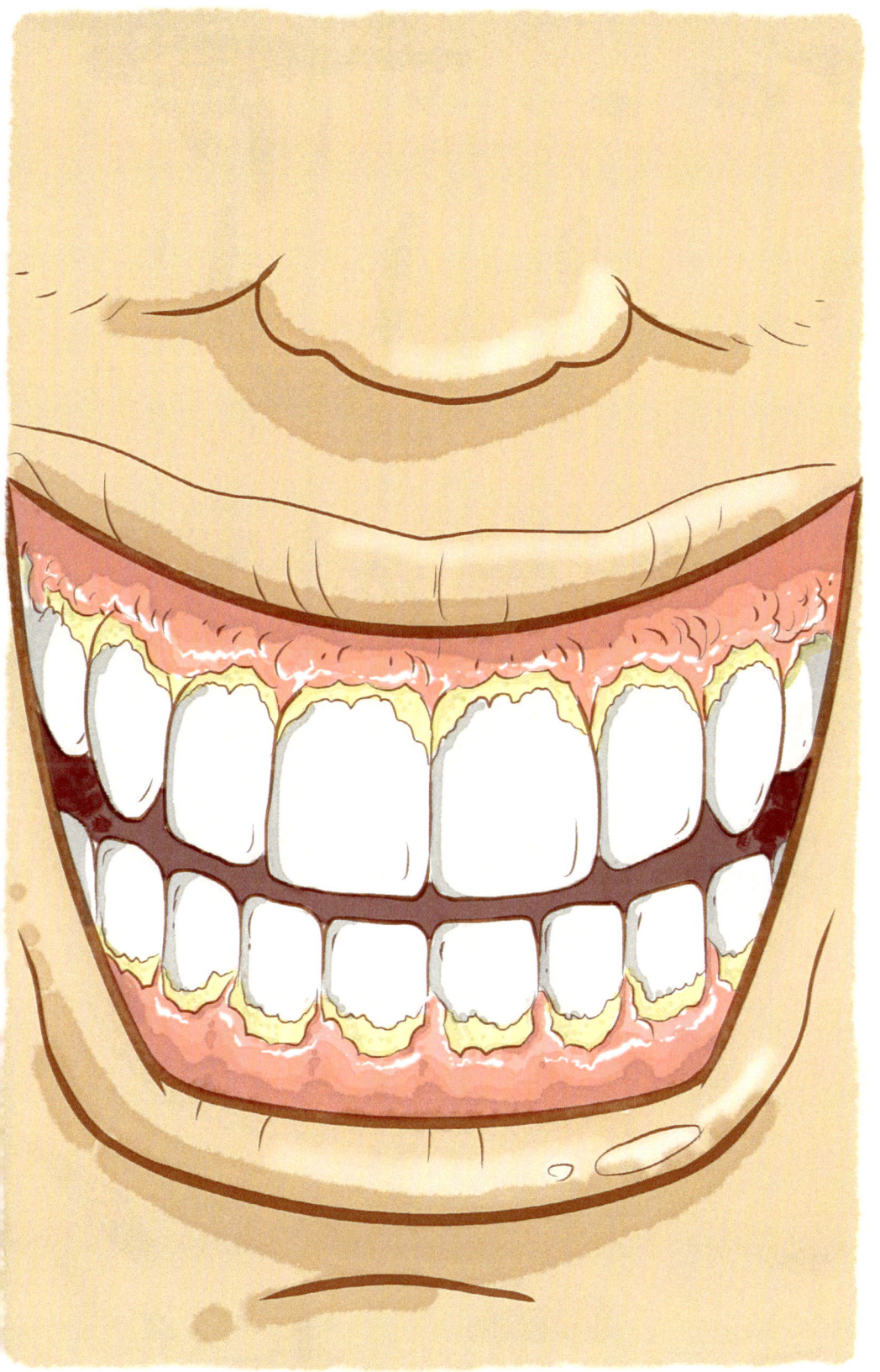

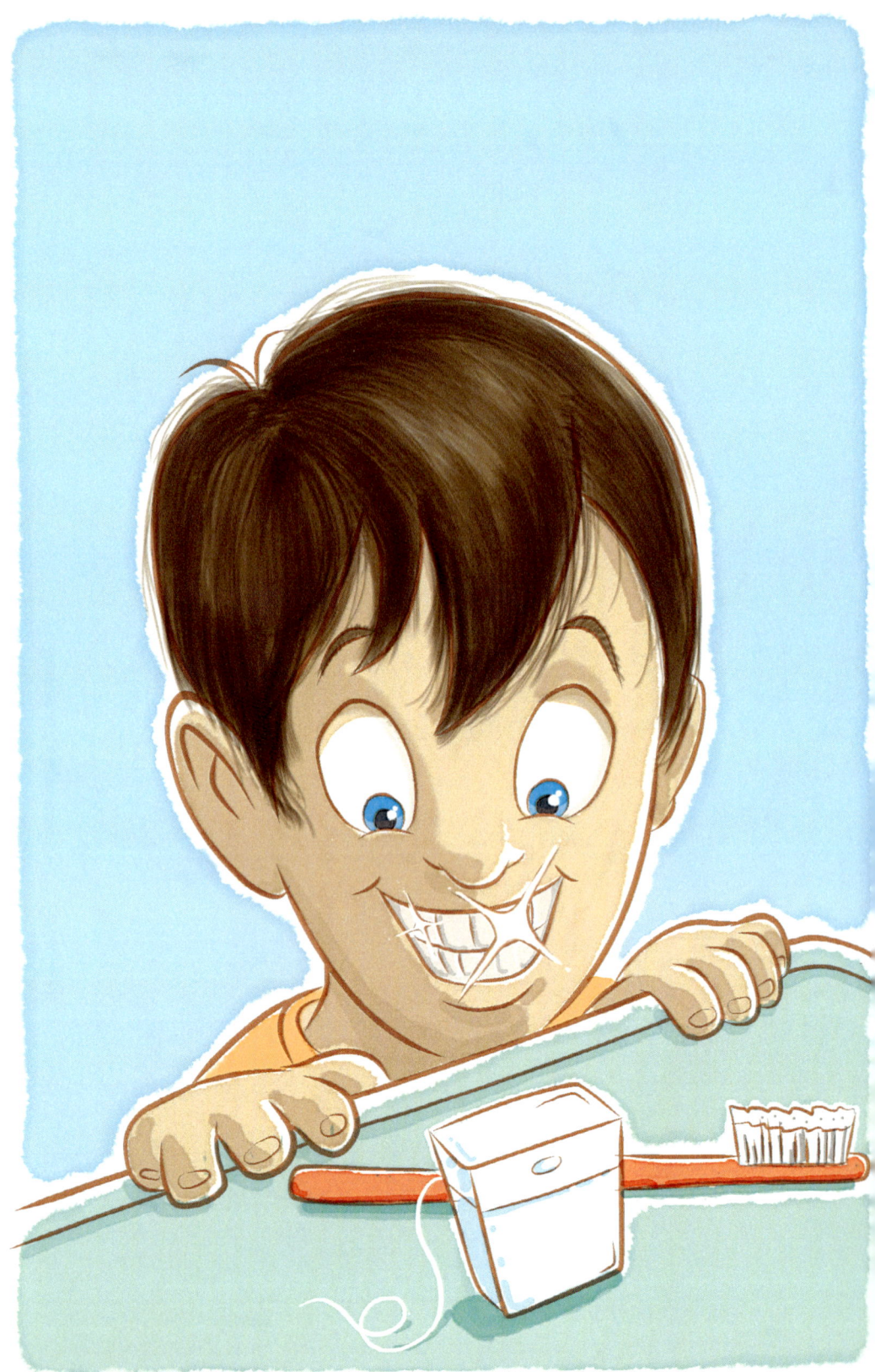

"It's true!" Dr. Tony said. "If you don't brush your teeth for a few hours, you can scrape your fingernail on your teeth and that white or yellow gunk you find is worm poop! We also call it *plaque*. This plaque is gross and makes your breath stink. It can cause holes in your teeth called cavities, and your gums could become red, swollen, and bleed easily. If your gums get too bad, your teeth could become loose and either fall out or have to be pulled out. I have seen teenagers who needed to have all of their teeth taken out and wound up with false teeth."

"I don't want false teeth like my grandma!" Joey said firmly.

"I don't blame you, Joey," Dr. Tony said. "The good news is that plaque can be removed with regular brushing and flossing. By brushing your teeth at least twice a day and flossing once a day, you can remove most of the plaque. The plaque you miss will turn into something called *tartar*, a film that hardens on your teeth. It can only be removed by someone at a dental office called a dental hygienist, like the one that cleaned your teeth today, Joey."

"Is there anything else I can do to keep worm poop off of my teeth?" said Joey.

"To have the healthiest mouth, you need to eat plenty of fruits and vegetables," said Dr. Tony. "You also need to limit the amount of sugar you eat or drink, like the kind you find in candy and soda pop. If you do have a sweet treat, brush afterward to protect your teeth. Brush and floss every day and go for your cleaning and checkup at the dental office twice a year. By following this plan, you'll end up with healthy teeth with little or no cavities, healthy gums, fresh breath, and most importantly...

No Worm Poop on Your Teeth!"

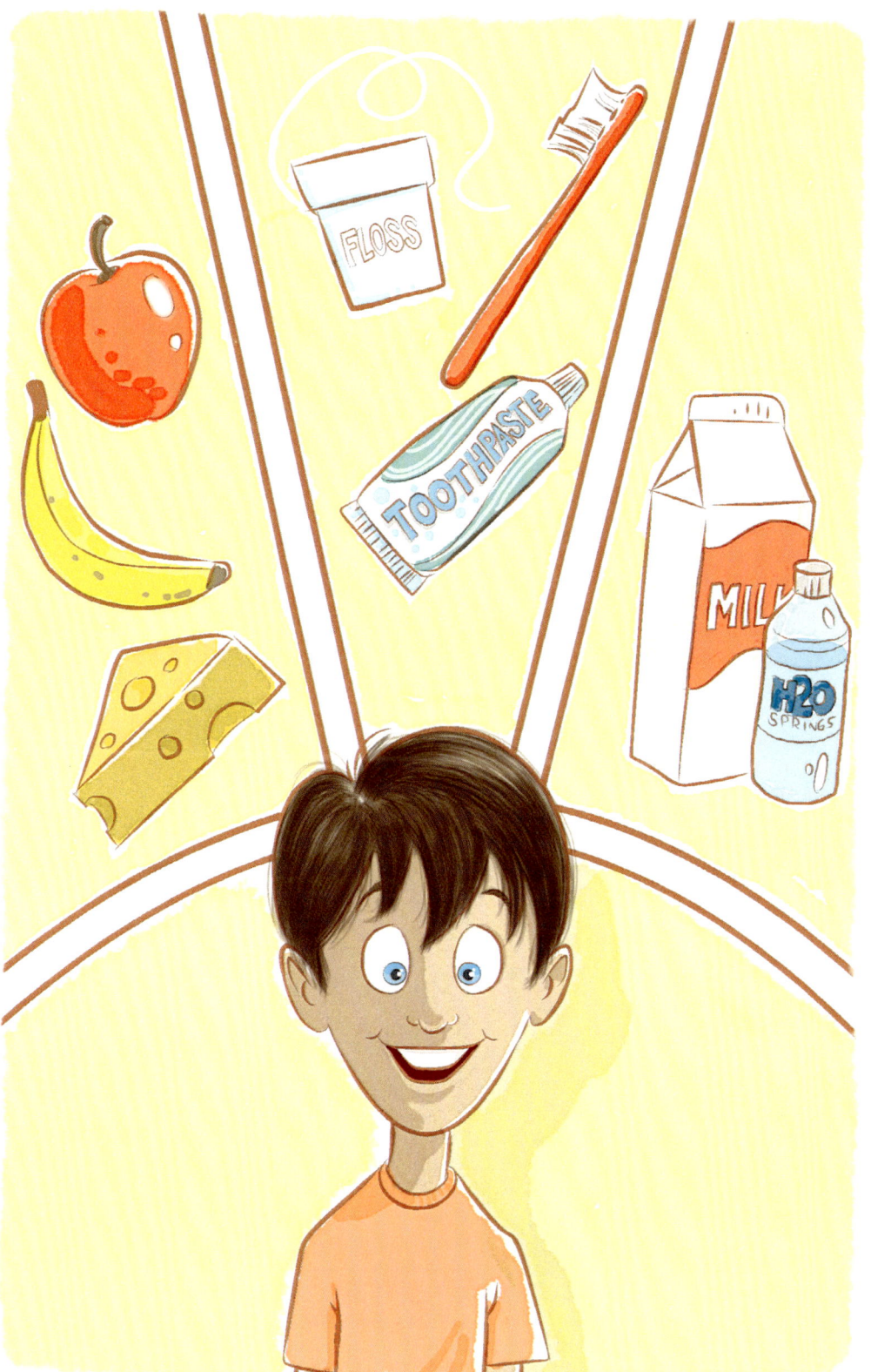

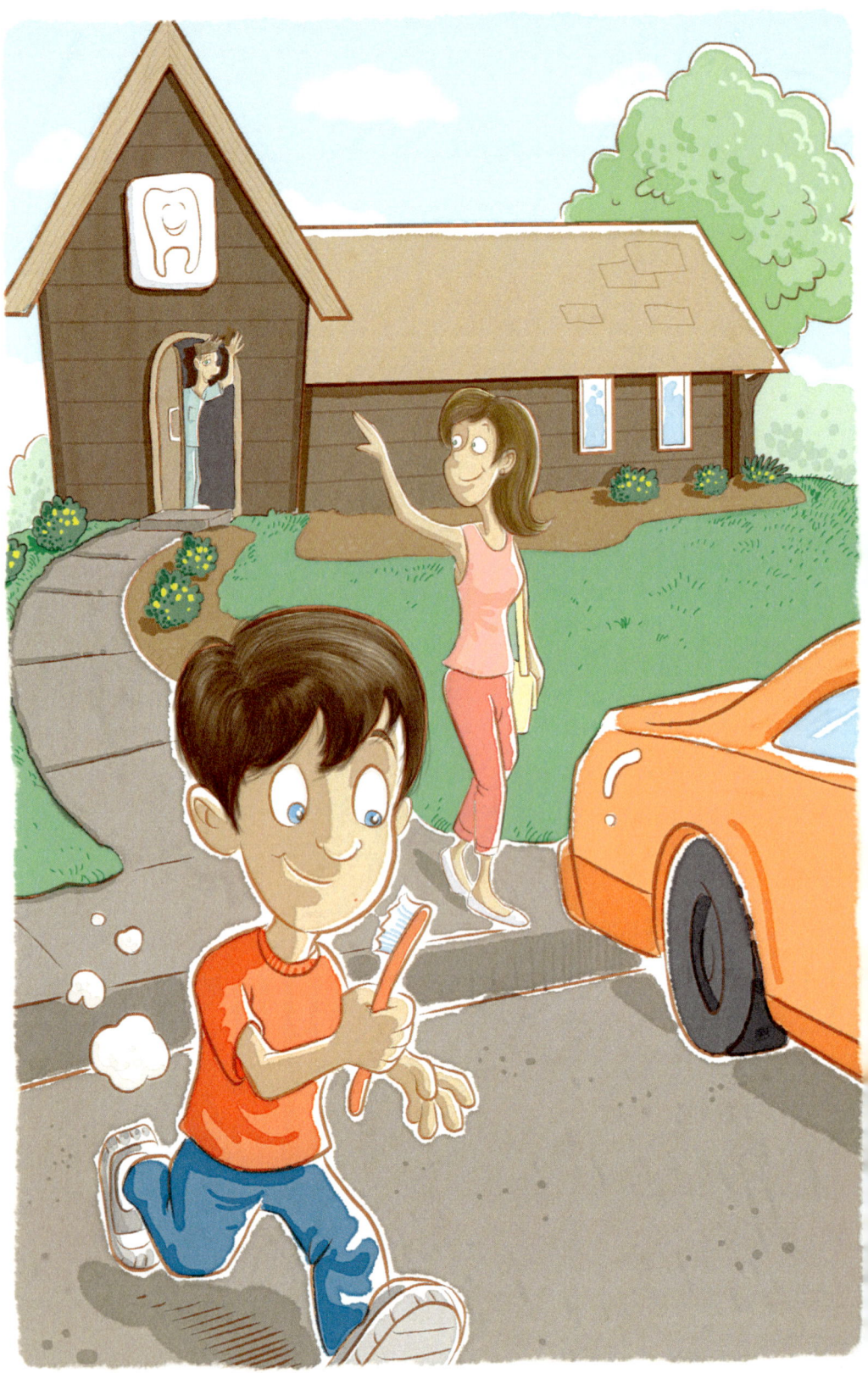

"Wow," said Joey. "I had no idea that was on my teeth. Can I go brush them right now?"

"You don't have to right now, Joey," Dr. Tony replied. "We just cleaned them for you. But when you get home, it's up to you to keep your mouth clean."

Joey left the office with his mom. They went home and Joey played for the rest of the day with his friends. When it came time for bed, Joey put his pajamas on and as usual, Kathy told him, "Joey, go brush your teeth before bed."

"I don't have to, Mom," said Joey.

"What do you mean, you don't have to?" asked Kathy.

Joey explained, "I don't have to because I already brushed and flossed. I'm not going to bed with worm poop on *my* teeth!"

"What are you talking about?" his mom asked.

"It's a long story," explained Joey, "I'll tell you later sometime."

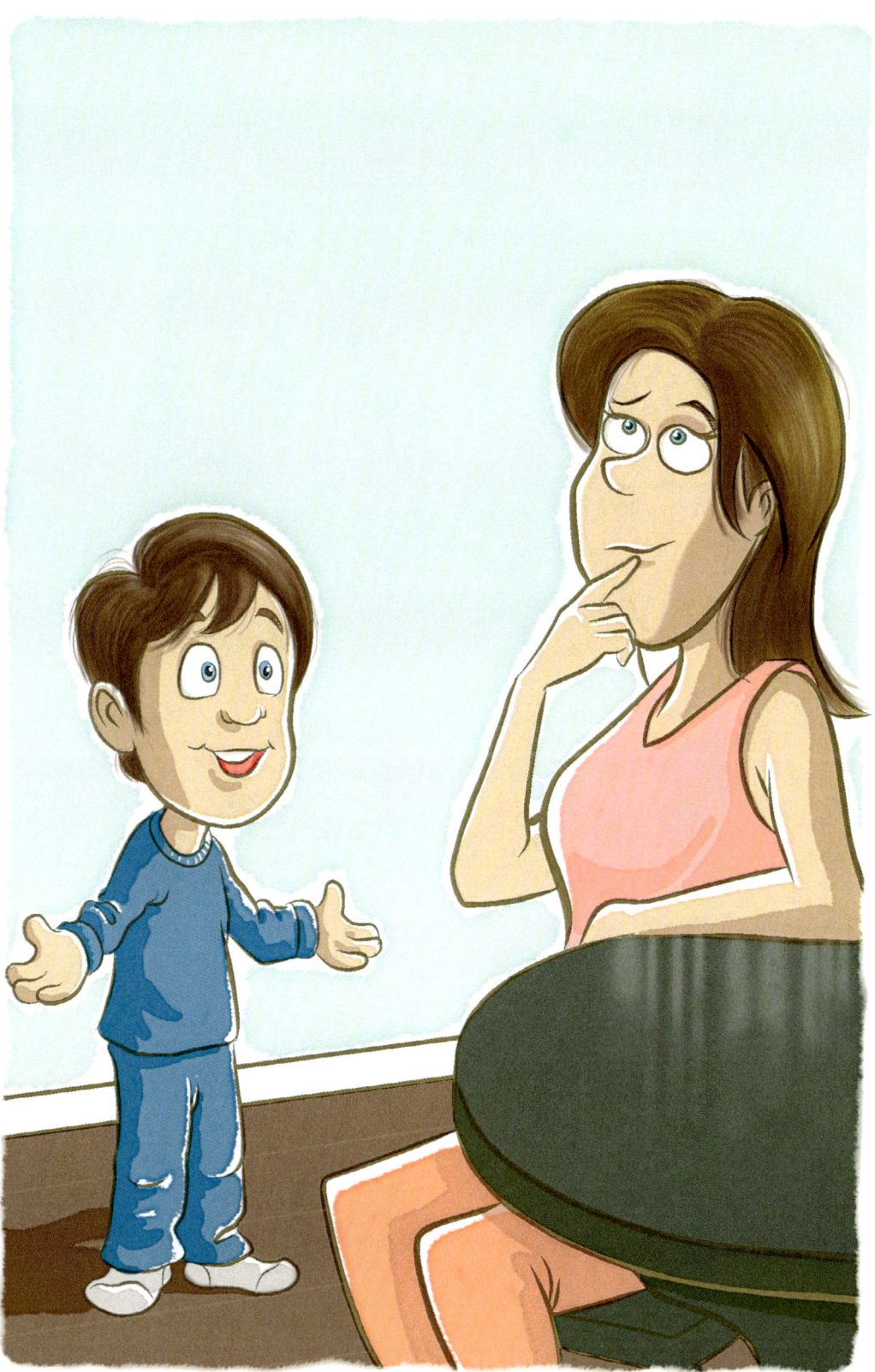

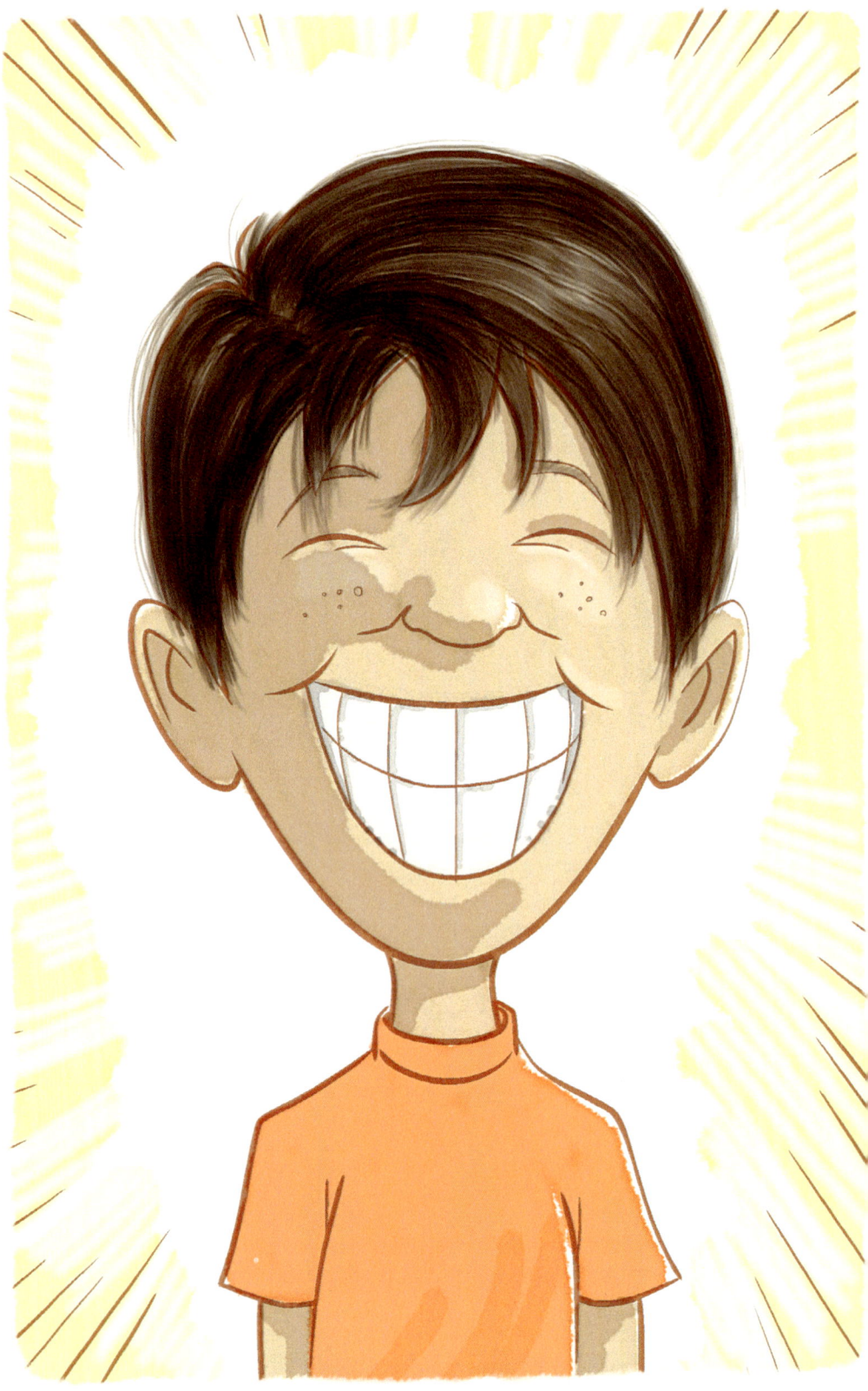

From that day forward, Joey took really good care of his mouth without having to be nagged. He didn't eat as many sweets and when he did he always went and brushed afterward. He didn't even give his mom a hard time when they went to see Dr. Tony for his cleaning and checkup. Joey was proud to show off how well he had been brushing and flossing and most importantly, how he had no...

Worm Poop on His Teeth!

Made in the USA
Middletown, DE
10 November 2016